LEARN HOW TO STOP SMOKING EASILY

This book reveals simple methods to
harness your willpower
and free yourself from nicotine addiction.

First printed March 2009

Reflex Communications Pty Ltd
P.O. Box 509
Biggera Waters
QLD Australia 4216

Learn how to harness your willpower
and stop smoking easily

Index

Chapter 1.	Why Stop	4
Chapter 2.	Honesty	9
Chapter 3.	Previous Attempts	12
Chapter 4.	Nicotine Addiction	17
Chapter 5.	Willpower	20
Chapter 6.	Strategy	23
Chapter 7.	Plan	31
Chapter 8.	Going Forward	39
	Interesting Items	42

Chapter 1.

Why stop?

Before you begin to think about how to stop smoking you must first think about why.
Why stop?
It is a simple question but the answer is quite complex. If it is to stop from dying, you would have already stopped. If it was to stop from smelling terrible you would also have stopped before now, the same goes for saving money, emphysema, getting fit, my family want me to, I hate it, I don't want my legs amputated, I'll do it for the kids etc. The fact is that you need to stop smoking so that you can have control of your life. You will never have control if you are addicted to nicotine. Cigarettes will always control you, you will spend your last dollar on cigarettes, you will go out in the middle of the night in winter for cigarettes, you will lie to your family and create arguments just to be able to smoke. You will plan cigarettes into holidays, meetings, car trips, dinners and everything else that forms part of your life.

This is a terrible way to live, there is a much happier and easier way to live, it doesn't cost you money, it doesn't rob you of self esteem, it doesn't harm your health and it brings you closer to your family, that's right, it is living without cigarettes. You don't need to worry about having that extra packet in the car, you don't need to worry about the thought of smoking until you choke to death, you can lead a life

where you no longer think of cigarettes at all.
There is an easy way to do this and it is within everybody's grasp. Willpower is the answer but there is a secret. Willpower doesn't mean going cold turkey and hoping for the best, it doesn't mean locking yourself away from the world and suffering indescribable agonies on your own, it doesn't mean battling everyday for the rest of your life knowing that every time you smell a cigarette you will be tormented into relapse. It doesn't mean going without until you find yourself alone where you can finally sneak in a cigarette without the stress of being discovered. It simply means stopping without the use of drugs, hypnosis or replacement therapies of any kind.
Don't be terrified.
I understand that this thought alone may make you want to have a cigarette or maybe two, how frightening. It actually isn't difficult at all, it's simple and you can learn the way to do it successfully. It does help to think of all the benefits of stopping but don't confuse these with the one reason that will actually make you stop.

Lets look at some of the benefits for not smoking

1. It would be nice to not smell terrible when you hug a loved one.
2. It would be nice to finish a meal and sit at the table talking to your family or friends instead of leaving to have a cigarette.
3. It would be nice to not cough, splutter, wheeze and gasp for air every time you have a good laugh.
4. It would be nice to not spend your last ten dollars until payday on cigarettes.

5. It would be nice to stay indoors in winter instead of freezing through a cigarette in the wind, rain or snow again and again and again.
6. It would be nice not to litter the planet with cigarette butts, it is disgusting trying to lay a picnic blanket in the grass or a towel on the sand at the beach just to find a half dozen discarded butts buried in the grass or sand.
7. I would be nice to be able to run and play with your children without having to stop for a cigarette or stopping because the blood no longer circulates to your legs properly.
8. It would be nice to give somebody a lift in your car without having to apologize for the horrible smell and the layer of ash that covers everything.
9. It would be nice to not be the person that stinks up the entrances of buildings and gets the evil eye from non smokers.
10. It would be nice to not be pitied by healthy people when you break into an involuntary coughing fit.
11. It would be nice not to have stained teeth and fingers and cigarette burns on your property.
12. It would be nice to not have to stand amongst the pack of smokers trying to rush in a last minute cigarette before a flight or meeting or anything else.

The benefits for not smoking could go on and on and on for pages and pages, but the benefits for smoking are zero, there is not one single benefit. Some might try to argue that the benefit is relaxation, non smokers can relax without having a cigarette or a cigar. Others might argue that it helps to make them think clearly. Well if this were true everybody with an important role in life such as brain surgeons, space shuttle pilots and life guards would be smoking non stop. Imagine scientists and doctors trying to find a cure for cancer by sitting around smoking all day so that they could think clearly about the research. The truth is nobody needs a cigarette to think clearly. These are simply arguments your mind uses to keep you feeling good about smoking, they are neither true nor valid. You could relax and think clearly before you started smoking so logically, when you stop you will still be able to relax and think clearly. No, there is not one single valid benefit to smoking. You began creating these excuses when you started smoking, your mind stored them away and used them whenever appropriate. How many times have you said, "I actually enjoy a cigarette after a meal", we have all said it and convinced ourselves it could be true. The same goes for, "I only smoke socially" or "I just like one at the end of the day," these sayings and many others are the things we gradually force ourselves to believe simply to justify the fact that we smoke. You cannot possibly enjoy choking down poison that you know is killing you under any circumstances, you have just lost that element of control that allows you to say no.

Regaining that element of control in your life will give you back self esteem, fitness, financial control, time, quality of life, social health, functioning taste buds and personal power – All of these and more were taken away one by one by cigarettes. One by one you began to use and believe the little one liners that keep you smoking, they calm me down, they pick me up, they help me sleep, they keep me awake, they stop me overeating, they're great after a meal, they help me relax, they help me focus.

There are so many one liners at your disposal to help you feel good about smoking. You do want control of your life back, that is why you have tried to stop before and are trying again now. Confidence, health and happiness all come from the one single, powerful step of regaining control.

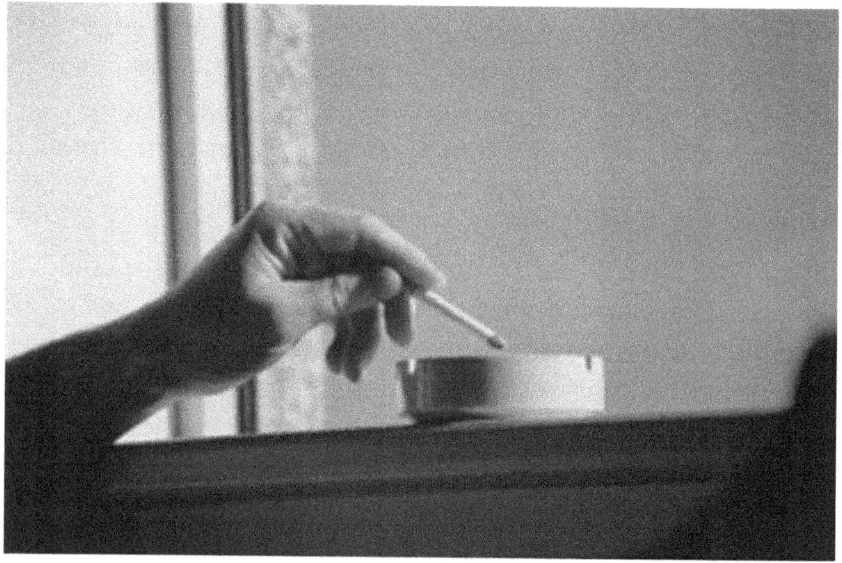

Chapter 2.

Honesty - A solid foundation

As the first step to successfully stopping smoking you must start with honesty. This is not the time to lie to yourself or others. You need to know that you are addicted to nicotine and know that you truly want to stop smoking, not because your husband or wife wants you to or you need to save money, but because you want your life back - control of your choices, inner strength and self esteem. These are the things you will get back, these are the things you are missing to certain degrees and these are the things you lie to others about in order to protect yourself. You will lie to people to protect yourself from them thinking that you are weak or not committed, or that you are selfish or hopelessly addicted. You will lie because it seems easier to lie and try again tomorrow than to disappoint your spouse, children or family. Honesty and humility are fundamental to the success in this willpower program. If you start with these two core elements you will succeed regardless of what methods you have tried and failed at.

I know, I have failed at every single method that I had tried until I understood where I was going wrong.

Each time I failed and most times I lied to my family and often my friends about the success I enjoyed, whilst still sneaking off when ever I could for a quick smoke. I would take longer to come home to enjoy a last cigarette and even start arguments at times just to be able to leave and have a cigarette in peace. I would go on errands that I would normally leave until the next day and insist on going alone just so I could have one more cigarette. The point is that I didn't admit I was addicted and had no plan to combat the fact that nicotine would make me lie to everybody I cared about including me, simply so that I could continue smoking. So first things first, admit you are addicted, concede that you will lie about the addiction given the chance and create opportunities to lie to conceal your addiction. Know that without any doubt you do want to stop smoking despite the fact that you may be scared about life with out cigarettes. It's alright if you are scared about stopping smoking, if you have smoked for a long time and cigarettes have formed a large part of your daily life, it can be a frightening concept. Even if you don't think you can do it you must know that you want to stop smoking more than anything else and cigarettes will make you lie to everybody to protect yourself. Once you do this you will have a true and solid foundation on which to base your strategy. You will be able to identify the traps you set for yourself and understand why you do it and how to combat it.

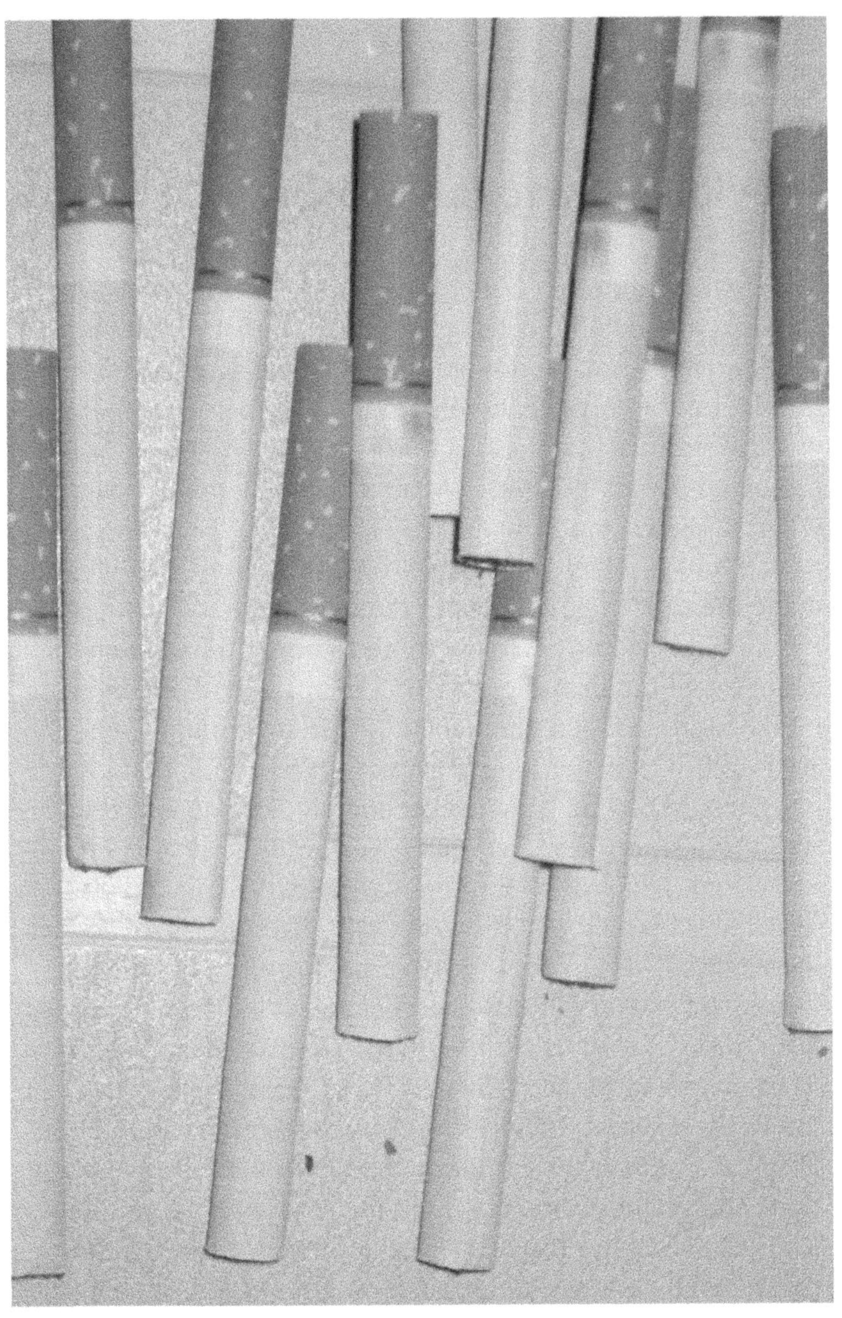

Chapter 3.

Previous attempts to stop.

Try to think about your previous efforts to stop, what went wrong and when did it go wrong. I know that often when I tried to stop smoking, I would renege on a promise to stop that I had with myself. I would opt for reducing the number of cigarettes despite the fact that just a few hours ago I promised myself this time I would do it. By this I mean when it got too hard I would say to myself, "I will buy a packet and just have one and throw them away, that will make it easier to go the rest of the day without cigarettes", I assumed it would be easier to go to none from one so the next day would be easier to stop. Then I would tell my wife I only had one cigarette and she would be proud of me, after all it was better than twenty or thirty. Then the next day I would buy another packet and smoke one and keep about five since it seemed that I was going to just have one a day for a while. Funny thing was I always smoked all five. Then I would tell my wife I only had one again so that she wouldn't think I was weak or be disappointed in me. The next day I would buy a packet but this time not throw them away, now I would have about five again and again lie to my wife. Before I knew it I was smoking in secret and lying about it. Other times I would accept a cigarette from a friend foolishly thinking that it would ease the stress of stopping. Unfortunately it led me straight back into the lying and smoking ritual I performed every time I tried to quit. This put enormous pressure on both my family and

me individually. If my family tried to talk about it, I would be allusive and suggest that talking about it stressed me out and made me want to smoke. This would enable me to avoid disclosing any level of my smoking or in turn blame them for making to hard to not smoke.
I would go to extreme lengths to disguise the smell or blame other smokers for the smell on my clothes. I used to stop on the way home and wash the smell of cigarettes from my face and hands with baby wipes then wash the smell of baby wipes off with clean water. The truth always came out in the end and I would justify the failure with some stressful event that made it impossible to stop. The truth is that I always had a reason at the ready:

1. I cannot give up in winter
2. I cannot give up in summer
3. I will do it next month
4. I just need to prepare mentally
5. After this project at work
6. When we go on holidays
7. After New Year
8. After my birthday

There was always an excuse not to stop immediately. Despite my list of excuses I always wanted to give up. I tried everything, I tried and failed at: hypnotism 3 times, Zyban twice, nicotine patches 5 times, nicotine chewing gum 5 times, mouth rinses twice, herbal cigarettes once, plastic nicotine infusers twice and acupuncture twice and meditation. Each time I failed and each time I lied about my failure for as long as possible, once the lies went on for almost three months before I was discovered.

In order to succeed you must understand that smoking nicotine is an addiction not a habit. You may do things that create patterns to your nicotine intake but it is still an addiction. If smoking every time you had a cup of coffee was a habit then not drinking coffee or tea for a week should cure the habit, but that never happens. In fact stopping anything you do when you smoke just makes you form new patterns to associate with smoking. Anything at all, so long as you keep smoking. This scenario makes the addiction seem less significant than it really is, until you notice that a new pattern always emerges to keep you smoking and eventually the old patterns creep right back in and often you are left smoking more than you previously did.

Your mind will always try to convince you that you are not addicted or justify your behavior. If you only smoke a few cigarettes a day you convince yourself that you need not give up now, you can do it any time. If you are smoking a lot, your mind will terrify you of the consequences of quitting just so that you never ever try to go without cigarettes for very long. This is what addiction to nicotine does, this is not what habits do. This is not a flaw in your brain. In your mind you are dealing with the short term problem of nicotine withdrawal and choosing to deal with the long term problems like health, financial and social issues at a later date. First things first, one step at a time in your mind, this is very natural.

This is also a key to understanding how to beat nicotine. If you concentrate on the short term issues you can never get to the long term issues because the short term issues arise over and over and over day after day after day.

Nicotine withdrawal – Have a cigarette, Nicotine withdrawal – Have a cigarette. Each time you have a cigarette it loads you up with nicotine enabling the withdrawal to happen, load up – withdraw, load up – withdraw, cigarette after cigarette, day after day, month after month, year after year. You should consider for a moment that if you don't load up with nicotine again you withdraw only once until the withdrawal is complete. However if you load up on nicotine over and over then you withdraw over and over. This means that the last cigarette you had is actually causing the next bout of withdrawal, and if you don't have another cigarette you will not have another withdrawal. Withdrawal is not a life long suffering, it is simply coming down from the last cigarette and it lasts only as long as there is nicotine in your system. Nicotine can only last in your system for about three days. Not only is it only three days but on the third day the nicotine level is so low that it is not really able to influence your thought patterns

As you begin this program you will be full of nicotine and have very little control over your life, towards the end of day one you will have significantly less nicotine in your system and as a result will have more control. Day two will see your nicotine level drop even further and your control level even higher Day three will see you in complete control and nicotine will no longer be a part of your life.

The graph on the following page explains this very simply.

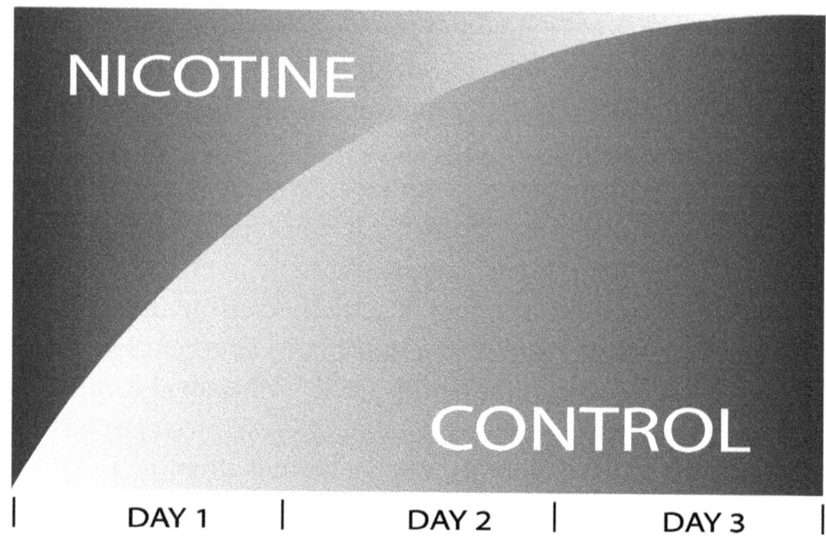

Day by day, control replaces dependence and your strength and resolve increases.

You cannot possibly beat nicotine addiction unless you know the time for you to stop smoking is NOW and you are prepared to do ANYTHING to succeed.
You must be aware that you need to stop smoking so that you are once again in control of your life. Every decision you make will be absolutely your own and you will not be influenced by cigarettes. You will no longer make sure you have enough cigarettes to get through a trip or make sure you have a cigarette to wake up to or that you have enough money to buy the next packet of cigarettes.
You must be honest about your addiction, the level to which you are addicted and the way addiction makes you do things you would not normally do. You must be humble in your admission, you are addicted to a drug. You must be determined to succeed.

Chapter 4.

Nicotine Addiction

You may have seen an ad on TV showing how the monsters in your brain march around and go crazy if they are deprived of nicotine so you have to give them nicotine to satisfy them. This is simply not true, it is a marketing campaign for nicotine, whether it be patches, chewing gum or some other replacement therapy. If you have two sugars in your coffee and you wanted to stop having sugar, switching to tea would not help, you actually have to stop the sugar. Nicotine is the same. You are not addicted to cigarettes - you are addicted to nicotine so why go from cigarettes to nicotine patches or nicotine gum, you actually have to stop the nicotine from entering your system to kick the addiction.

Try to remember the last time you went to bed and slept eight hours. When you woke up, did you have to be rushed to hospital because of your withdrawal. After you have been on a long haul flight for 10, 12, 14 hours or more hours did you have to have an ambulance meet you at your destination to revive you or inject you with a drug to calm you until you could have that next cigarette? Of course not. Not once have you ever needed any sort of drug, resuscitation or medical intervention because of nicotine withdrawal. If you did, you would be terrified of going to sleep. The reason for not needing medical attention is that nicotine addiction is more mental problem than physical.

Although there is a real physical addiction, there really is no physical pain at all, just a slight discomfort when you stop smoking, it is only your mind that knows you are not smoking. Your mind knows you are addicted to nicotine and will ensure that you do whatever you need to so that you can continue to smoke therefore avoiding the discomfort of withdrawal. This means your mind will create the arguments so you can smoke. Your mind will make it ok for you to lie so that you can continue to smoke. Your mind will make it ok to sneak off and hide away while you secretly have a cigarette. Your mind will even make it ok to have two in a row from time to time in case you have been without for a while. In fact the entire battle to stop smoking is in your mind. That doesn't mean it is imagined, it means you are battling yourself. That's why you feel like you're going crazy and you think you need a cigarette. You don't feel like you are going crazy from the pain, but mentally you cannot think of anything other than cigarettes. If you want to successfully stop smoking you need to have common sense answers to the need for nicotine. You need valid responses for yourself when your mind begins arguing for the short-term problem of nicotine withdrawal. All of the failures and relapses in the past have been because of your lack of mental preparation to deal with the withdrawal from nicotine. You know this to be true, that is why you fear going without nicotine, not because of the physical pain you will suffer but because of the mental anguish and battle you will have to face with yourself.

It is your preparation for this battle alone that will determine your success.

In the past you have actually been using your willpower when you attempt to quit, unfortunately you have been using it to keep yourself smoking not for stopping. In the face of all evidence, health, financial, social, environmental and the fact that you actually desperately want to stop, you continue to permit yourself to smoke. Not only do you permit yourself, but you actually create opportunities through lies, arguments and deception to allow yourself to smoke, and where possible blame anything or anyone else other than yourself.

Now that is willpower.

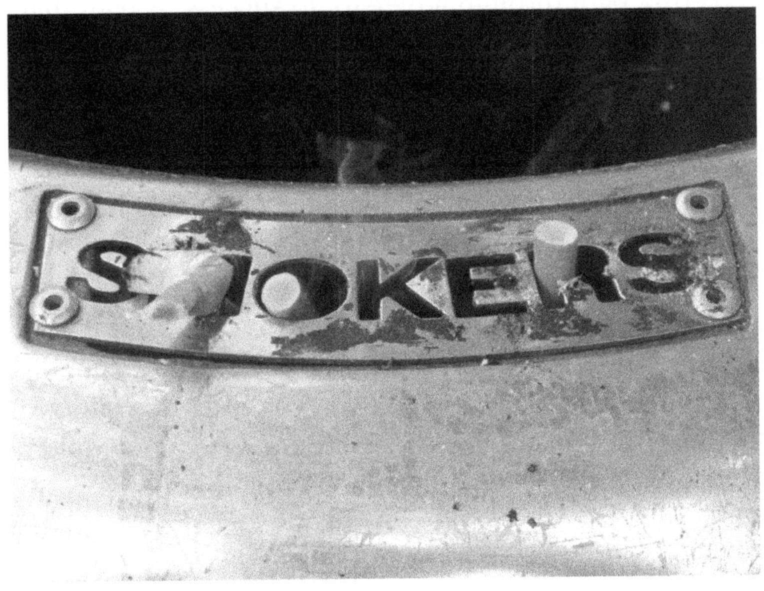

Chapter 5.

Willpower

Willpower is a powerful tool to ensure that you achieve your goals. Willpower is not hoping for the best, willpower is not giving it a try, willpower is not thinking you might just do it this time.

Willpower is a successful strategy to defeat the negative thoughts and mental war you are about to have. Willpower is about being prepared for the arguments, the self-defeating logic, the permission to fail, the excuses and the lies. Willpower is knowing what you want and setting an unwavering path through adversity to success. A path that you can easily follow to achieve your goal. Previously you have used strategies to continue smoking regardless of whether you knew that was what you were doing. Now you must turn these around so your strategies are to stop. It is that simple. Previously when you have failed it is because your mind has had better strategies to keep you smoking than it has to allow you to stop. This means your willpower is working perfectly, just for the wrong cause. Your desire, reasons, excuses and opportunities to smoke have been honed and reinforced over and over, day after day and year after year. But you are not a fool, if you were you would not want to give up, you would be happy to kill yourself slowly one cigarette at a time until your final wheezing breath.

So you know that cigarettes are bad and that you don't want to smoke, now you must make your arguments to stop smoking more compelling than your arguments for smoking.

Your arguments must be real, factual and common sense, this way there can be no valid argument against them. This is how willpower works, it is not magic, it is common sense and an unwavering desire to succeed. It is a belief in the truth and a respect for yourself. It is knowing what you want and knowing how to get it. The only easy and painless way to stop smoking is to use willpower, this is how you can stop without an ongoing fight in your mind. Using willpower this way will allow you to stop and never want or feel like a cigarette again. Every day will be as if you never smoked. It is simple and without a doubt the most effective way to stop. The beauty is that if you have tried every other way that you can think of and have failed every time, it is because of your will to smoke. Your willpower works perfectly, in fact it is extremely strong. Now you just need to turn it to what you actually want in the long term, not what you think you need to do to solve a short term problem.

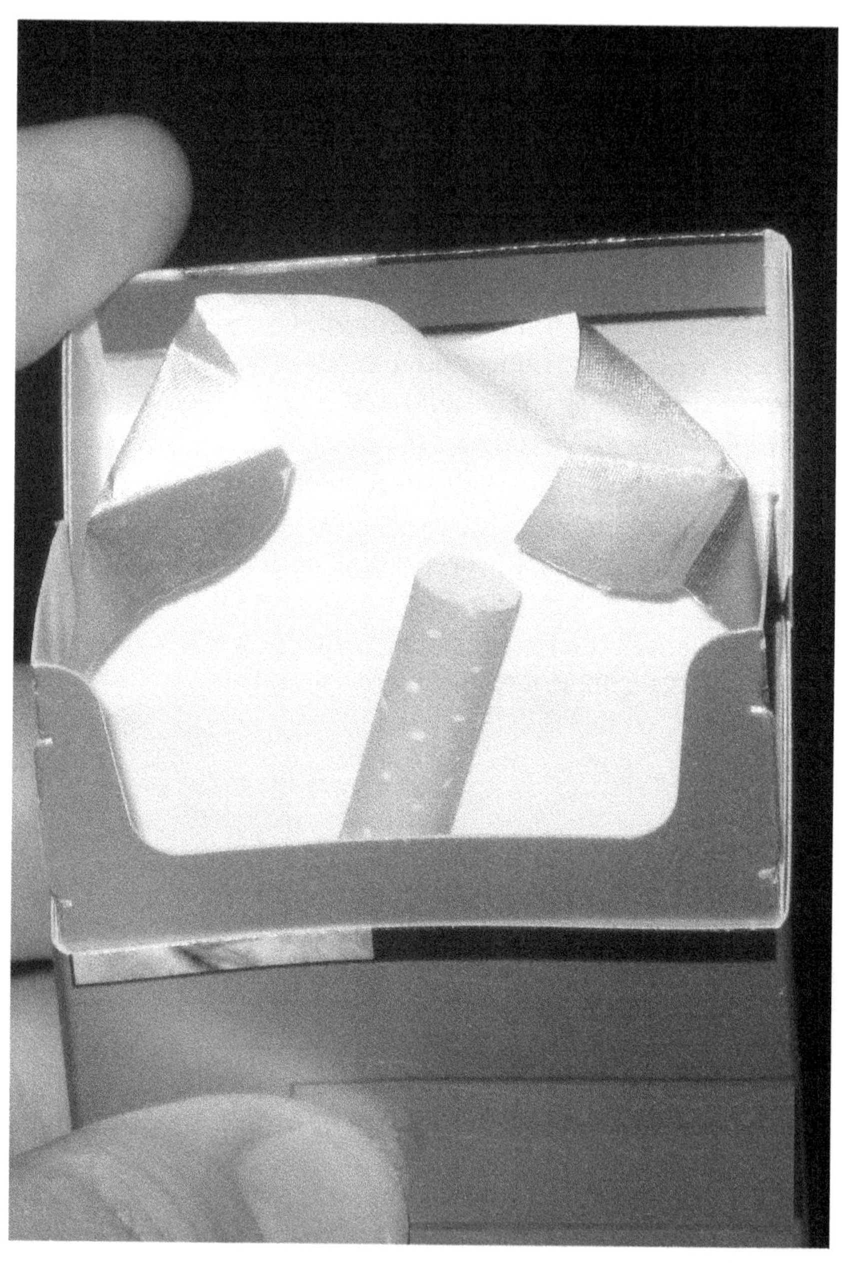

How much time have you spent ensuring you don't run out?

Chapter 6.

Strategy

Now is the time to get your strategy in place for the next three days. I say three days because after three days there is barely a trace of nicotine left in your body and the fourth day will see you completely nicotine free. That's right its only three days and you will never smoke again, and the best bit is that you get to sleep for about one third of that time. Let's say you start on a Thursday night, when you wake up on Friday morning you will already be almost half way through the first day. By the time you go to bed again you will be one third of the way to never smoking again. When you wake up on the second day you will be almost half way through the entire program and by the time you go to bed that night you will be two thirds through the program and the worst of the battle will be well and truly over. When you wake on the third day you will be transformed and have a completely new sense of power over your own destiny, on the third day you will know without a doubt that you will never smoke again.

It sounds really easy doesn't it, that's because it really is that easy if you prepare to use your willpower for yourself and not for cigarettes and take advantage of key achievements to boost your morale and your determination.

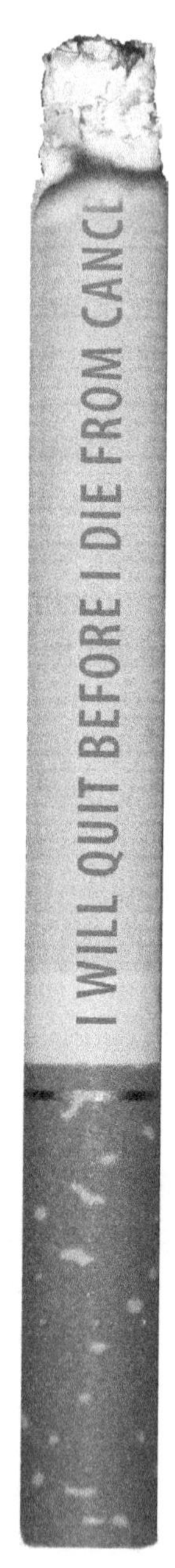
I WILL QUIT BEFORE I DIE FROM CANC

Key factors

The first thing you must understand is the feeling you get when you think you need a cigarette, it is not you at a weak point, it is actually you winning. As the amount of nicotine in your body diminishes your body begins to return to a normal – non addicted state, exactly the goal you are aiming for. What you have previously seen as you suffering a craving is actually your body running out of nicotine and returning to normal. That is the feeling of you succeeding and each time you feel it, it turns a little more into a strength, a feeling that the addiction is dying. Previously when you felt this craving returning to normal was not the desired result so a cigarette was smoked to increase the level of nicotine. When you see the withdrawal as a path to success instead of failure it actually works for you. Withdrawal becomes part of your strategy to stop instead of the addictions key method of getting you to smoke again. When you feel what you think is a craving, you **MUST** say to yourself.

NO, I DO NOT WANT A CIGARETTE.
THIS FEELING IS MY BODY RUNNING OUT OF NICOTINE AND RETURNING TO NORMAL.
THIS IS EXACTLY WHAT I WANT.
THIS TIME THE ADDICTION WILL DIE AND I WILL WIN.

Try to imagine the nicotine draining away as your body returns to normal and you regain control, every craving sees the nicotine diminishing further until it barely exists

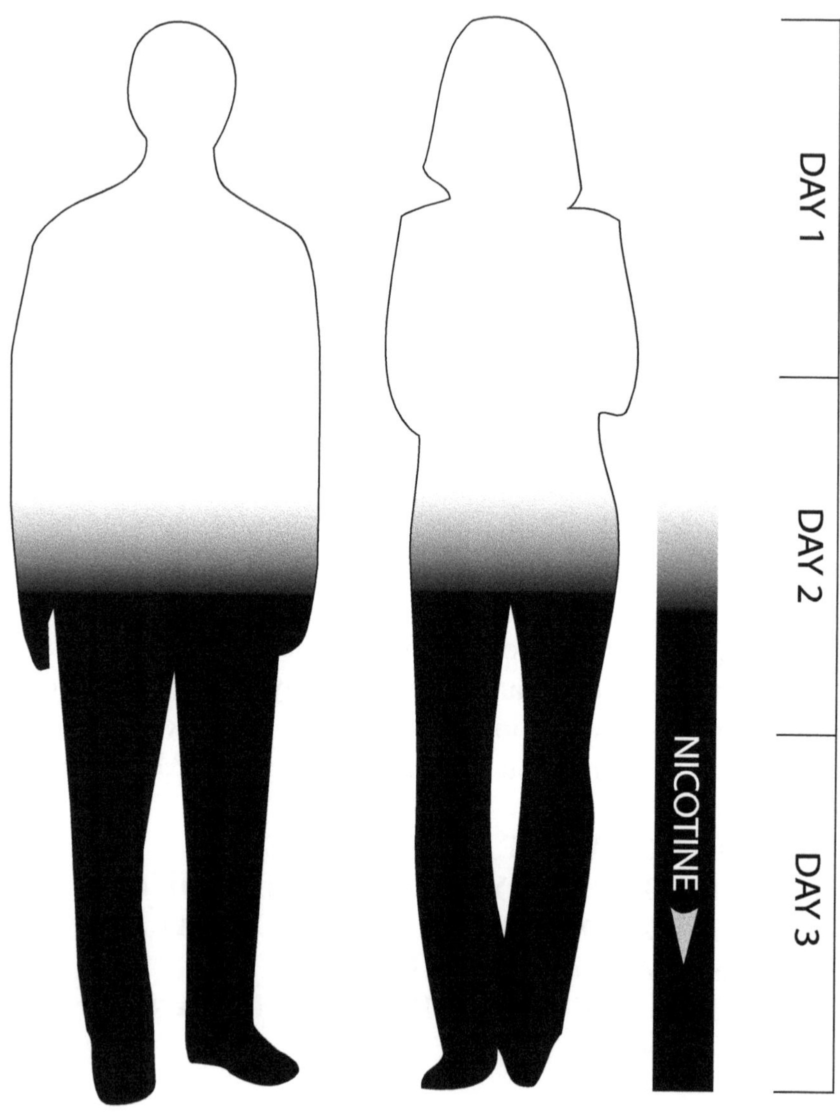

Remember the goal is to rid yourself of nicotine, nicotine is the problem, day by day you will feel stronger as you feel yourself becoming nicotine free.

Understand that you are stopping smoking not giving up smoking. Giving up suggests that you are sacrificing something in order to be a non-smoker. The truth is that you gave up your freedom and choices when you started smoking. So make certain to always say I have stopped smoking, not I have given up or I am giving up. Think of smoking as a start and stop process. This means when you light a cigarette you start smoking and when you extinguish it you stop smoking. This means after every cigarette you stop smoking, then you are a non-smoker until you start again with the next cigarette. When you have your last cigarette at night you are a non-smoker until you start again the next day. All you have to do then is when you stop smoking, don't ever start again. Never have a cigarette again, because the moment you do you are a smoker again. The thought of the start/stop process is very powerful and will help you enormously in the first two days. This will help you remember that you have stopped smoking and are not giving up.

Don't try and think that you are battling cigarettes for ever, hundreds and thousands of them for your entire life far into the future.
You actually only need to battle one cigarette.

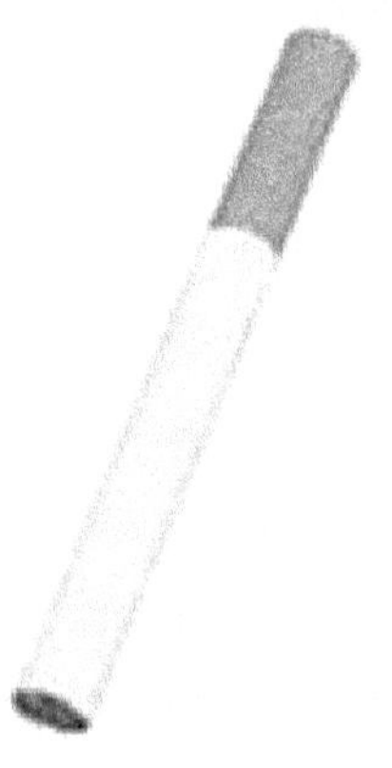

Next Cigarette

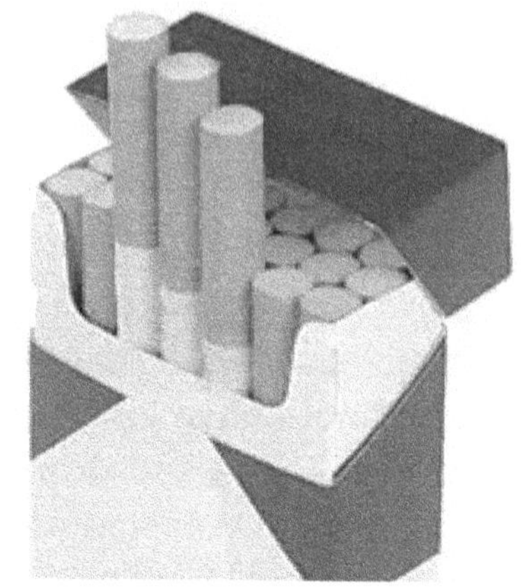

Cigarettes after the next one

The next one, that's all you need to fight, if you never have that one (next) cigarette you never have to worry about any of the cigarettes after that.
Affirmation statements are another powerful key factor to your success. These statements are actually the answers you will give yourself when your mind begins questioning the logic and your ability to stop. You must use these statements as arguments with yourself not as sweeping statements. They must form the basis of your mission, go over them again and again and say them aloud not just in your head. Say them aloud with strength and conviction. You must believe them above everything else, after all you know them to be true.

When your mind says to you, mmm I feel like a cigarette.
You must say,
NO, NO I DO NOT FEEL LIKE A CIGARETTE, THAT IS THE LAST THING I WANT, THAT IS WHY I AM STOPPING, I HATE SMOKING, I HATE WHAT IT HAS DONE TO ME.

You must say this loud and emphatically, there is no room for weakness. This is an argument and you can and must win.

When your mind says to you, I'm going crazy, just one cigarette will make it easier to stop.
You must say,
NO, NO IT WILL NOT MAKE IT EASIER TO STOP, JUST ONE CIGARETTE IS HOW I FAIL OVER AND OVER AGAIN, I WILL NEVER HAVE A CIGARETTE. I HAVE STOPPED SMOKING AND I WILL NOT SMOKE AGAIN, THIS FEELING IS ACTUALLY MY BODY RETURNING TO NORMAL, THE NICOTINE ADDICTION IS DYING AND I WILL BE FREE.

When your mind says, mmm I can smell a cigarette, I would love a cigarette. You must say,
I STOPPED SMOKING BECAUSE I HATE SMOKING, I WOULD NOT LOVE A CIGARETTE, I DO NOT WANT A CIGARETTE, I WILL NOT HAVE A CIGARETTE, I WILL NEVER SMOKE AGAIN.

Make your own strategies. Think about the times you failed and be prepared to argue with yourself when those times arise. For example many people fail at social functions.

Be prepared, when somebody offers you a cigarette.

Refuse.
NO THANK YOU, I HAVE STOPPED SMOKING,
walk away and say to yourself:

I AM SO HAPPY I DON'T DO THAT ANYMORE, THAT'S NOT ME, I STOPPED SMOKING AND I WILL NEVER SMOKE AGAIN.

It helps to listen to the smokers coughing, wheezing and hacking through the event. Look at their stained fingers and teeth and the blanket of ash on them and the ground around them, smell the putrid stench of the smoke lingering on their breath and in their clothes when they walk past you and say: **I AM SO GLAD THAT IS NOT ME, I WILL NEVER DO THAT TO MYSELF AGAIN, I WILL NOT SMOKE, I REFUSE TO.**

You must understand how powerful each of these statements are. You must believe them and use them as the answers you seek. These are the keys to your willpower succeeding. Remember the battle is in your mind, it is not physical. The physical addiction is not even enough to wake you up at night, preparation mentally will ensure success.

You know what it is like arguing with somebody who will not change their mind no matter what happens. That is how you must be. Do not change your mind no matter what you hear, see or feel. You stopped smoking and that is that, you will not start again, ever.

Chapter 7.

Plan

Now is the time to choose the time to stop once and for all. Choose a day in the next day or two, not weeks away, not for a vacation or some other time when you are really putting it off. Choose a day in the next day or two. I chose a Thursday night and took the Friday off work as annual leave. I did this so that I could have three days clear,
amongst people that I wanted to benefit from me stopping. People who would share my happiness and help me with affirmation statements if I needed. I spoke to my family about my strategies and the way nicotine might try to cause trouble to allow me a reason to smoke, I spoke to them about ways to combat this if they saw it happening. Not getting drawn into arguments and reminding me that it is a battle between me and addiction and the withdrawal is my body becoming nicotine free. Exactly what I wanted. You should choose a time that makes sense for you and speak to your family. Knowledge and preparation will ensure your success. Before you go to bed at the beginning of this process dispose of all smoking paraphernalia ie, lighters, cigarettes. Sit down somewhere comfortable and have your last ever cigarette. As you smoke that final cigarette, think about what it is doing to you, what it has cost you over the years and whether you want to live without addiction or die addicted.
Understand that is the trade off, - **the addiction lives and you die or you live and the addiction dies.**

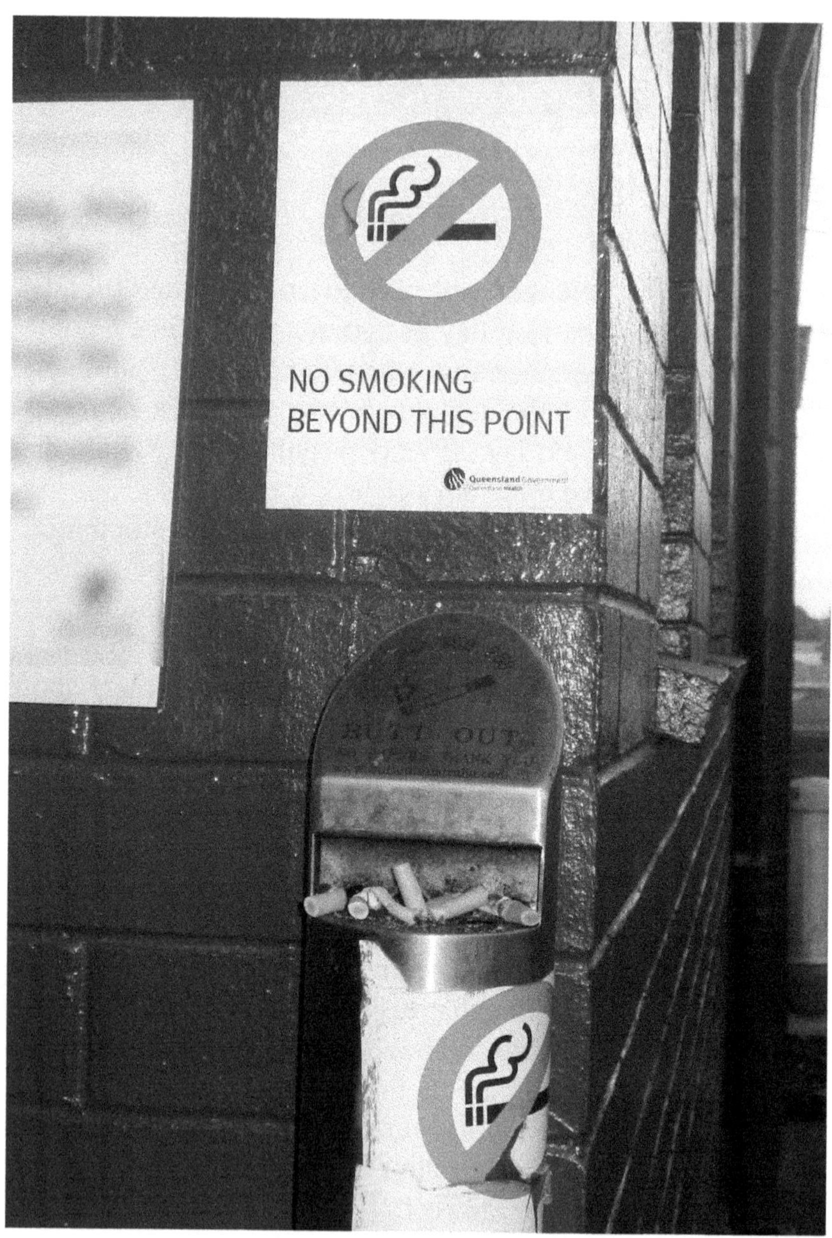
NO SMOKING
BEYOND THIS POINT
Queensland Government

Take a shower and put your clothes in the washing machine. Do some light exercise, some stretching, deep breathing or similar. This is not for fitness, this is to help get some good clean air in your lungs before you go to bed. Take some deep breaths while you are lying in bed and taste the clean air. Say to yourself:

THIS TIME I WILL SUCCEED, I WILL NEVER SMOKE AGAIN, I HAVE STOPPED SMOKING AND I ABSOLUTELY REFUSE TO START SMOKING AGAIN. I WILL LIVE AND THE ADDICTION WILL DIE.

When you wake up in the morning, say to yourself:

I STOPPED SMOKING YESTERDAY AND ALL I NEED TO DO IS NOT START AGAIN, I REFUSE TO SMOKE,

I DO NOT WANT TO SMOKE, I WANT TO WIN.

I WILL NOT HAVE THE NEXT CIGARETTE, THIS WILL BE MY LAST WITHDRAWAL.

Start the day with a healthy light breakfast, do not clog yourself with greasy breakfast and coffee. Have something you can enjoy the taste of without being stuffed to the gills. Really enjoy the taste. After eating take some deep breathes and enjoy the freshness of the air.

If you feel the need for a cigarette, understand that it is not a nicotine craving, it is actually your body returning to a nicotine free state. Soon this feeling will actually turn into a strength to help you remain nicotine free. When you feel this feeling, enjoy it. It means you are winning the battle. It means the nicotine addiction is dying and you are emerging from its grip - fresh, free and alive.

As you go through your day, use the affirmation statements whenever you need to, when you see somebody smoking out

the front of a building, say to yourself:
I AM SO HAPPY THAT IS NOT ME ANYMORE.
When you see somebody driving in their car with a cigarette hanging from an open window, say to yourself:
IT DOESN'T MATTER HOW FAR YOU HANG IT OUT THE WINDOW YOUR CAR WILL STILL SMELL LIKE AN ASHTRAY, I AM SO GLAD THAT'S NOT ME.
When you see somebody smoking near a child, say to yourself:
I AM SO GLAD I STOPPED, I WILL NEVER SMOKE AGAIN, I AM FREE.
When you are with your family or friends tell them how proud of yourself you are. Please be aware that they will be proud of you also but really they don't care if you smoke or not. They love you regardless. They will be happy if you stop smoking, but ultimately it is your life and only you will be really proud of yourself and ecstatic that you stopped, this can only be your victory. Do some more light exercising or stretches, get into bed and take some more deep breaths.
When you go to bed at the end of the first day, say to yourself:
I DON'T BELIEVE I REALLY DID IT, ONE WHOLE DAY WITHOUT SMOKING, I HAVE DONE THIS WITHOUT TAKING DRUGS OR LYING OR CHEATING. I AM REALLY GOING TO DO IT THIS TIME. I AM SO PROUD OF MYSELF.
Don't be afraid to be really proud of yourself.
When you wake on the second day you truly can be proud of yourself, you are half way through the program. The second day is easier because you already know you can go a whole day. You have to be prepared for the battle still using your

affirmation statements with conviction, you must believe in the strength you get from them.

The arguments your mind will put forward will be a little different today.
BE PREPARED

Your mind might say things like, congratulations you went a whole day, celebrate with a secret cigarette, nobody will know. If that happens, you must say to yourself:
NO, NO WAY WILL I HAVE ANOTHER CIGARETTE FOR ANY REASON WHAT SO EVER, I WILL NOT SMOKE AGAIN. I REFUSE.
Your mind might say, its still difficult, you want a cigarette, if you have one now that's only one every two days, that's better than 25 a day and you can slowly go down from there. Do not fall for these tricks say to yourself:
NO, I DO NOT WANT TO SMOKE, I AM SO GLAD I STOPPED AND I WILL NOT START AGAIN. I WILL NOT SMOKE. I REFUSE.
Follow the same affirmations as yesterday when you see smokers or smell them. Each time you must argue in your favour emphatically. You must say:
I WILL NOT SMOKE, I REFUSE, I WILL NEVER SMOKE AGAIN, I AM SO GLAD THAT'S NOT ME, I AM A NON SMOKER, I AM FREE.
At the end of the second day tell yourself again how proud you are that you really, honestly did it. Tell your family how proud you are of yourself. Again they will be proud of you too, but they can never really understand the victory you have had and you cannot expect them to. This is your victory and yours alone to celebrate.

Before you go to bed the second night, again do some exercise or stretching, get some air into your lungs. Take some deep breaths in bed and taste the air. Surprisingly it really does taste better. Say to yourself:

I DID IT, TWO COMPLETE DAYS WITHOUT NICOTINE, I KNOW NOW I AM FREE, I WILL NEVER START SMOKING AGAIN.

On the third day when you wake up you can be sure that you are so close to complete freedom and control that you have no doubt you will not smoke. You can actually sense the victory. The third day there is so little nicotine in your body that it cannot generate any interest in smoking. The battle is now completely in your mind and you are already winning that battle. There is absolutely no need to smoke, the affirmation statements roll off your tongue without even thinking, you are a non-smoker.

Beware of the sneaky tricks your mind will use, things like – Congratulations you did it, now you know you can do it anytime, have a cigarette. You know you don't need them and can stop again anytime, even straight away.

You must say:

WHERE DID THAT COME FROM, GET OUT OF MY HEAD, THERE IS NO WAY I WILL SMOKE, I WILL NOT FALL FOR THESE TRICKS, I WILL NOT SMOKE, I REFUSE, I WILL NEVER START SMOKING AGAIN.

Stick with the affirmation statements. Their power will have increased three fold by now. One statement will keep the thought of cigarettes out of your head for hours and hours, you will be happy and feel strong about not smoking. You must be able to laugh when you do things like go to pick up

your cigarettes from where you used to keep them. This will happen from time to time when you do things mechanically. For example, a month after you stop smoking you might pick up your car keys from your desk and then go to get your cigarettes from where you used to keep them.
When these things happen, just laugh and say:
THAT'S RIGHT I DON'T SMOKE, I STOPPED SMOKING AND WILL NEVER START SMOKING AGAIN.

When you go to bed at the end of the third day, again do some light exercises and deep breathing. Know that when you wake up you will have won, the battle will be over and you will be the victor. You should be extremely proud of yourself. There is no more nicotine in your body and the affirmation statements have become the powerful tools for success that will keep you smoke free for the rest of your life. All you have to do is never start again, never.

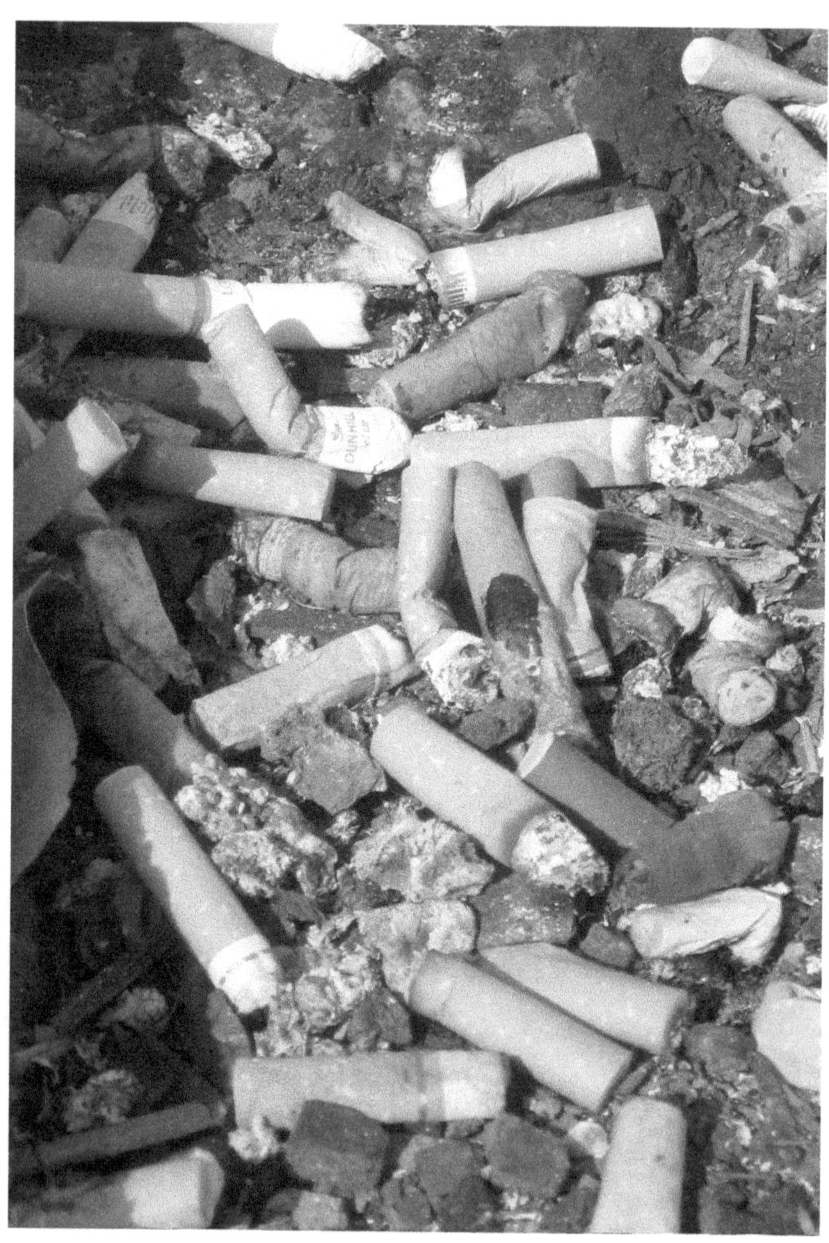

You will not be a part of this anymore.

Chapter 8.

Going Forward

So now you have control of your smoking after all these years. What do you do now and how do you make sure you stay free of nicotine. How do you avoid becoming one of those people that stop for three months and then start again? The people that start smoking again never mean to start again, they simply fall for one of those arguments like, Congratulations! You did it. Now you know you can stop anytime. Just have one now then don't have anymore. Unfortunately having just one is actually starting again, the very thing you must avoid at all costs. You must never under any circumstances start smoking again.

Have you ever watched a movie where there is a heroin addict and they go through a terrible ordeal in rehab to come out clean. The first time they find themselves in a situation from their past were heroin is available to them, we sit back and watch hoping they don't take heroin, knowing full well if they do just a little it is all over for them. Begging to the screen for them to not do it, just to get away..... THAT IS YOU, *(just with nicotine instead of heroin)* when you find yourself being led into something you do not want.... GET AWAY AND DON'T DO IT.

You can start a light exercise program and begin to get fit again, eat well and watch your weight. Clean your car and keep it clean. Clean up the cigarette butts that are in your garden or around your house. You must always use the affirmation statements. Use them at every opportunity, it will get less and less until you actually go months without even thinking about it. You can count the days that you are free of nicotine with pride, 4 days, 10 days 15 days. Days turn into weeks, three weeks, four weeks, six weeks. Weeks turn into months, two months, three months, six months. Then you stop counting and wait for one year to roll around. You must never forget that smoking is a start and stop process. If you stop for six months and fall for a sneaky mind trick that came out of nowhere, like -

Its six months now, you are free, you're at a party just have one, it doesn't mean you have to have another tomorrow...

Then you go right back to the start. That's right, you cannot have one cigarette without going right back to the start and going through it all again.

YOU MUST NEVER START AGAIN

Not for a party, not because your best friend had a baby, not a cigar for New Years, not for any reason at all. If you never start again you will always be free and always be a non-smoker. I cannot emphasise this enough, it is paramount to your success that you understand this. If you have a cigarette or cigar for whatever reason then you are once again a smoker and will have to go through the entire program again or as many smokers will testify, keep smoking for years. Do not fall for the mind traps you set for yourself, it is very easy to say:

NO, I WILL NOT SMOKE, I REFUSE.

And you will stay smoke free.

When you have reached this point it is actually easier to not smoke than it is to smoke, to not smoke you just have to not have a cigarette. To smoke you have to find a cigarette, buy one or get one from a friend. You have to actually put it in your mouth and light it, then suck the poison into your lungs.

You have to suffer the humiliation of letting yourself down and quite often you have to start lying to your family again. There goes your health, money and social life – there goes your control.

It is far easier to just not start again. Stay alert and stay clean and free.

Remember when you smoked saying the phrase that every smoker says to themselves and their friends, -

I wish I never started or why did I ever start smoking or if I had my time over I would never start smoking. Well this is your chance, this is your time over and your chance to never start, grab hold of it.

Congratulations, good luck and remember,

NEVER START AGAIN.

Some interesting data about smoking

The amount of people that die from smoking related diseases in America per year is the similar to a Jumbo Jet crashing and killing everybody onboard twice a day, every day 365 days a year.
In Australia alone, it is similar to a bus crashing and killing everybody on board every day 365 days a year.

Every day more than 3000 children smoke their first cigarette.

90% of all smokers began smoking as children.

Smoking reduces life expectancy on average by about 8 minutes per cigarette, or 4 hours per pack of 30.

If you smoke a packet of 30 cigarettes a day for 10 years you will inhale approximately one kilo of tar.

105 Billion cigarettes are sold each week around the world, that's approximately 10 Million per minute.

In 1996 Australian school children smoked more than 370 Million Cigarettes.

Smoking kills more people in Australia than the total number killed by alcohol, drugs, murder, suicide, road crashes, rail crashes, air crashes, poisoning, drowning, fires, falls, lightning, electrocution, snakes, spiders and sharks.

In Australia in 1986, the following body organs were removed from humans because of cancer caused by smoking:
521 lungs, 148 gullets, 71 tongues, 221 voice boxes,
82 stomachs, 40 pancreases, 68 wombs, 85 bladders 115 kidneys and 161 miscellaneous body parts.

Around 140 Australian non smokers die each year from lung cancer caused by breathing other people's smoke.

Tobacco related deaths annually;
1.2 million China, 438,000 America, 650,000 Europe, 45,000 Canada, 300,000 Russia, 140,000 Germany, 800,000 India, 86,500 England, 66,000 France, 50,000 Spain, 49,000 South Korea, 50,000 Iran, 34,000 Egypt, 13,000 Scotland, 6,000 Ireland, 6,000 Cuba, 19,000 Australia, 22,000 Saudi Arabia.

In 1996 Phillip Morris spent more than $3 Billion advertising and promoting cigarettes.

In 1998 470 billion cigarettes were smoked in the USA producing in excess of 176 Million pounds of discarded filters all containing known carcinogens that easily leech into the environment when in contact with water, most smokers discard butts directly into the environment. Globally the figure is more than 2.1 Billion Pounds (over 950,000 tons) of filters. These figures do not include remnant tobacco weight. Cigarette filters are made of Cellulose acetate fibers that can take 10 years to degrade. World wide Trillions of butts accumulate in streets and gutters leeching toxins into our streams rivers and oceans through storm water.

www.ingramcontent.com/pod-product-compliance
Ingram Content Group UK Ltd.
Pitfield, Milton Keynes, MK11 3LW, UK
UKHW020229250726
13967UKWH00001B/270